Title: "Pawsitively Delicious: Homemade Dog Food Recipes for Healthy Canines"

Chapter 1: Understanding Canine Nutrition

- Exploring the nutritional needs of dogs
- Importance of balanced meals for optimal health
- Common misconceptions about dog food ingredients

Chapter 2: Homemade Vs. Commercial Dog Food

- Pros and cons of homemade dog food
- Understanding commercial dog food labels
- How to transition your dog to homemade food safely

Chapter 3: Kitchen Essentials For Homemade Dog Food

- Essential tools and equipment
- Safe food handling practices
- Tips for storing homemade dog food

Chapter 4: Building Balanced Meals For Dogs

- The role of protein, carbohydrates, fats, vitamins, and minerals
- Recommended ratios for different life stages and breeds
- Choosing the best ingredients for your dog's needs

Chapter 5: Meaty Marvels: Protein-Packed Recipes

- Chicken and Sweet Potato Stew
- Beef and Barley Casserole
- Turkey and Vegetable Stir-Fry

Chapter 6: Carb Creations: Wholesome Grain And Vegetable Dishes

- Brown Rice and Lentil Medley
- Quinoa and Spinach Delight
- Pumpkin and Oatmeal Bake

Chapter 7: Healthy Treats And Snacks For Happy Pups

- Peanut Butter and Banana Biscuits
- Carrot and Apple cakes
- Frozen Yogurt Drops

Chapter 8: Special Diets And Considerations

- Recipes for dogs with allergies or sensitivities
- Homemade diets for senior dogs
- Tips for overweight or underweight dogs

Chapter 9: Meal Planning And Batch Cooking

- Creating a weekly meal plan for your dog
- Batch cooking and freezing homemade dog food
- Time-saving tips for busy pet parents

Chapter 10: Beyond The Bowl: Supplementing Your Dog's Diet

- Adding fresh fruits and vegetables
- Incorporating supplements for joint health and shiny coats
- Homemade remedies for common health issues

Acknowledgement:

I would like to express my heartfelt gratitude to everyone who contributed to the creation of this book.

First and foremost, I extend my deepest appreciation to

my family for their unwavering support, encouragement, and understanding throughout this journey. Your love and patience have been my greatest source of strength.

I am immensely grateful to my dedicated team of editors, researchers, and advisors for their invaluable assistance and expertise in bringing this book to fruition. Your commitment to excellence and attention to detail have enriched every page of this manuscript.

I extend my sincere thanks to the veterinary professionals and experts who generously shared their knowledge, insights, and guidance, enriching the content of this book and ensuring its accuracy and relevance.

I also want to acknowledge the countless dogs and their loving owners who inspire us to prioritize their health, happiness, and well-being. Your stories and experiences have shaped the content of this book and underscored the importance of homemade dog food and holistic pet care.

Lastly, I extend my appreciation to the readers who have embarked on this journey with me. Your interest in providing the best care for your canine companions motivates me to continue advocating for their health and welfare.

Thank you to everyone who contributed to this project in ways big and small. Your collective efforts have made this book possible, and I am deeply grateful for your contributions.

With heartfelt thanks,

[Kenneth Christopher]

Foreword:

In writing this book, I am reminded of the profound bond between humans and dogs, a relationship that spans millennia and transcends language and culture. Dogs have been our companions, protectors, and confidants throughout history, enriching our lives in countless ways.

In recent years, there has been a growing awareness of the importance of holistic pet care and the role of nutrition in promoting the health and well-being of our canine companions. As pet owners, we have a responsibility to provide our dogs with the best possible care, including nutritious and balanced meals that support their unique dietary needs.

In this book, we explore the world of homemade dog food, delving into the nutritional requirements of dogs, debunking common misconceptions about commercial pet food, and providing practical tips and recipes for preparing wholesome meals at home. From protein-packed stews to nutritious grain and vegetable dishes, you'll find a variety of delicious and nutritious recipes to nourish your furry friend from nose to tail.

I am deeply grateful to the author for undertaking this important endeavor and for sharing their knowledge and expertise with pet owners everywhere. May this book serve as a valuable resource for dog lovers seeking to provide the best possible care for their beloved companions.

Warm regards,

[Kenneth Christopher]

Chapter 1: Understanding Canine Nutrition

Dogs, our faithful companions, rely on us to provide them with the nutrition they need to thrive. In this chapter, we delve into the fundamentals of canine nutrition, shedding light on the essential components that make up a healthy diet for our four-legged friends.

Diving into the World of Dog Nutrition:
- We explore the unique dietary requirements of dogs, from puppies to seniors, and how these needs vary depending on factors such as breed, size, and activity level.
- Understanding the role of macronutrients (proteins, carbohydrates, and fats) and micronutrients (vitamins and minerals) in supporting your dog's overall health and well-being.
- Unveiling the importance of water in your dog's diet and how to ensure they stay adequately hydrated.

Separating Fact from Fiction:
- Addressing common misconceptions about dog nutrition, such as the notion that all fats are bad for dogs or that grains are inherently harmful.
- Debunking myths surrounding homemade dog food and its feasibility in meeting your dog's nutritional needs.

Navigating Commercial Dog Food:
- Deciphering dog food labels and understanding what ingredients to look for (and avoid) when selecting commercial dog food for your furry friend.
- Exploring the pros and cons of various types of commercial dog food, including kibble, wet food, and raw diets.

Taking a Holistic Approach:
- Emphasizing the importance of a balanced diet in promoting overall health, longevity, and vitality in dogs.
- Highlighting the significance of regular veterinary check-ups

and consultations with veterinary nutritionists to ensure your dog's nutritional needs are being met.

By gaining a deeper understanding of canine nutrition, you'll be better equipped to make informed decisions about what to feed your beloved canine companion, setting them on the path to a healthier and happier life.

Exploring the Nutritional Needs of Dogs

Dogs, like humans, require a balanced diet to support their growth, energy levels, and overall well-being. Understanding their nutritional needs is crucial for providing them with the best care possible. Here's a breakdown of the key nutrients that dogs require:

1. Protein:
   - Essential for building and repairing tissues, muscles, and cells.
   - High-quality protein sources include meat, poultry, fish, eggs, and legumes.
   - Adequate protein intake is especially important for active dogs, growing puppies, and pregnant or nursing females.

2. Carbohydrates:
   - Provide a source of energy for dogs, fueling their daily activities.
   - Complex carbohydrates such as whole grains (e.g., brown rice, oats, barley) and vegetables (e.g., sweet potatoes, peas, carrots) are ideal choices.
   - Carbohydrates also contribute fiber, aiding in digestion and promoting gastrointestinal health.

3. Fats:
   - Serve as concentrated sources of energy and are essential for the absorption of fat-soluble vitamins (A, D, E, and K).
   - Healthy fats include those from animal sources (e.g., chicken fat, fish oil) and plant sources (e.g., flaxseed oil, coconut oil).
   - Omega-3 and omega-6 fatty acids play a crucial role in maintaining healthy skin, coat, and immune function.

4. Vitamins and Minerals:
- Play various roles in maintaining overall health, including bone and teeth development, immune function, and metabolism.
- Vitamin-rich foods include fruits and vegetables, while minerals can be found in meats, grains, and dairy products.
- Ensuring a balanced variety of vitamins and minerals in your dog's diet is essential for preventing deficiencies and promoting optimal health.

5. Water:
- Often overlooked but arguably the most critical nutrient, water is vital for maintaining hydration, regulating body temperature, and facilitating digestion.
- Fresh, clean water should be readily available to dogs at all times, especially during hot weather or after exercise.

Meeting your dog's nutritional needs involves providing a balanced diet that includes a variety of protein sources, carbohydrates, fats, vitamins, minerals, and plenty of fresh water. Consulting with a veterinarian or veterinary nutritionist can help tailor your dog's diet to their specific requirements based on factors such as age, breed, size, and health status. By prioritizing proper nutrition, you can help ensure your dog lives a long, healthy, and happy life.
Importance of Balanced Meals for Optimal Health

Just like humans, dogs benefit greatly from a balanced diet to maintain optimal health and well-being. Here's why balanced meals are essential for your canine companion:

1. Nutritional Adequacy:
- Balanced meals provide all the essential nutrients in the right proportions to meet your dog's specific needs. This includes proteins, carbohydrates, fats, vitamins, and minerals.
- Each nutrient plays a vital role in various bodily functions, from supporting growth and development to maintaining immune function and overall health.

2. Weight Management:

- A balanced diet helps regulate your dog's weight, preventing obesity or undernutrition. Proper portion control and the right balance of nutrients can help your dog maintain a healthy body weight.

- Maintaining a healthy weight reduces the risk of obesity-related health issues such as joint problems, diabetes, and heart disease.

3. Energy Levels and Vitality:

- Dogs require energy to fuel their daily activities, whether it's running, playing, or simply lounging around the house. A balanced diet provides the necessary energy to support your dog's lifestyle and vitality.

- The right balance of carbohydrates, fats, and proteins ensures sustained energy levels throughout the day, keeping your dog active and engaged.

4. Digestive Health:

- A well-balanced diet promotes digestive health by providing adequate fiber for regular bowel movements and supporting a healthy gut microbiome.

- Proper digestion and nutrient absorption are essential for preventing digestive issues such as diarrhea, constipation, and gastrointestinal discomfort.

5. Strong Immune System:

- Balanced meals contain essential vitamins, minerals, and antioxidants that support a strong immune system. A healthy immune system helps your dog fight off infections and diseases, reducing the risk of illness.

- Nutrient-rich foods such as fruits, vegetables, and lean proteins provide the vitamins and minerals necessary for immune function and overall health.

6. Healthy Skin and Coat:

- Omega-3 and omega-6 fatty acids, found in balanced meals,

are essential for maintaining healthy skin and a shiny coat. These fatty acids help reduce inflammation, alleviate itching, and prevent dryness and flakiness.

- A balanced diet also ensures proper hydration, which is crucial for skin health and overall hydration.

By providing your dog with balanced meals tailored to their specific nutritional needs, you can help them live a longer, healthier, and happier life. Consulting with a veterinarian or veterinary nutritionist can help you create a customized diet plan that meets your dog's individual requirements and promotes optimal health.

Common Misconceptions about Dog Food Ingredients

Despite our best intentions, misconceptions about dog food ingredients can lead to confusion and misinformation. Here are some common misconceptions debunked:

1. "Grains are bad for dogs":
- While some dogs may have grain allergies or sensitivities, grains can be a valuable source of carbohydrates, fiber, and essential nutrients for many dogs.
- Whole grains such as brown rice, oats, and quinoa provide energy, fiber, and nutrients that contribute to a balanced diet.

2. "All fats are unhealthy for dogs":
- Fats are an essential component of a dog's diet, providing energy, supporting nutrient absorption, and maintaining healthy skin and coat.
- While excessive fat intake can lead to obesity, healthy fats from sources like fish oil, chicken fat, and coconut oil are beneficial for dogs in moderation.

3. "By-products are low-quality ingredients":
- By-products are often misunderstood and unfairly labeled as low-quality ingredients. In reality, by-products can be nutritious and provide valuable protein and nutrients for dogs.
- By-products include organs such as liver, kidney, and heart,

which are rich in essential vitamins and minerals that contribute to overall health.

4. "Raw food diets are inherently safer and healthier":
   - While some advocates tout the benefits of raw food diets for dogs, these diets come with risks such as bacterial contamination (e.g., Salmonella, E. coli) and nutritional imbalances.
   - Raw food diets may lack essential nutrients or be unbalanced, leading to deficiencies or excesses that can harm your dog's health.

5. "Natural and organic ingredients are always better":
   - While natural and organic ingredients may sound appealing, their quality and nutritional value vary. Not all natural or organic ingredients are superior to conventional ones.
   - What's most important is the overall balance and quality of ingredients in your dog's diet, regardless of whether they're natural, organic, or conventional.

6. "Homemade dog food is always safer and healthier":
   - While homemade dog food can be nutritious when formulated correctly, it requires careful planning and attention to ensure it meets your dog's nutritional needs.
   - Homemade diets may lack essential nutrients or be unbalanced, leading to deficiencies or excesses if not properly formulated.

By dispelling these common misconceptions, pet owners can make more informed decisions about their dog's diet, focusing on providing balanced meals that meet their nutritional needs and promote overall health and well-being. Consulting with a veterinarian or veterinary nutritionist can provide valuable guidance in selecting the best diet for your dog.

Chapter 2: Homemade Vs. Commercial Dog Food

When it comes to feeding your furry friend, you're faced with the choice between homemade and commercial dog food. In this chapter, we'll explore the pros and cons of each option to help you make an informed decision for your canine companion.

Homemade Dog Food:
Pros:
1. Control Over Ingredients: With homemade dog food, you have complete control over the ingredients that go into your dog's meals. This allows you to customize the diet to meet your dog's specific nutritional needs and preferences.
2. Quality and Freshness: By preparing homemade dog food, you can ensure the quality and freshness of the ingredients used. You can use fresh, whole foods without artificial preservatives or additives.
3. Tailored to Dietary Restrictions: Homemade dog food is ideal for dogs with food allergies, sensitivities, or specific dietary restrictions. You can easily avoid common allergens and customize the diet to accommodate your dog's unique needs.
4. Bonding Experience: Cooking for your dog can be a rewarding experience and a great way to bond with your furry friend. It allows you to show love and care through homemade meals made with affection.

Cons:
1. Time-Consuming: Preparing homemade dog food requires time and effort, including meal planning, shopping for ingredients, and cooking. It can be challenging to maintain consistency and variety in your dog's diet, especially for busy pet parents.
2. Nutritional Imbalance: Without proper knowledge and guidance, homemade dog food runs the risk of being nutritionally imbalanced. It's essential to consult with a veterinarian or veterinary nutritionist to ensure the diet meets your dog's

nutritional requirements.

3. Cost: Homemade dog food can be more expensive than commercial options, especially if you're using high-quality, organic ingredients. The cost of ingredients, supplements, and kitchen equipment adds up over time.

4. Potential for Contamination: Improper handling or storage of homemade dog food can increase the risk of bacterial contamination, leading to foodborne illnesses in dogs.

Commercial Dog Food:

Pros:

1. Convenience: Commercial dog food offers convenience and ease of use, requiring minimal preparation and storage. It's readily available in various forms, including dry kibble, wet food, and semi-moist pouches.

2. Complete and Balanced: Reputable commercial dog foods are formulated to meet the nutritional needs of dogs at different life stages. They undergo rigorous testing to ensure they contain the right balance of protein, carbohydrates, fats, vitamins, and minerals.

3. Affordability: Commercial dog food is often more affordable than homemade options, especially when considering the cost per serving and the time saved on meal preparation.

4. Long Shelf Life: Commercial dog food typically has a longer shelf life than homemade food, thanks to the addition of preservatives and packaging methods that maintain freshness and prevent spoilage.

Cons:

1. Lack of Transparency: Some commercial dog foods may contain low-quality ingredients, fillers, or artificial additives that provide little nutritional value. Reading and understanding ingredient labels can be challenging for pet owners.

2. Potential for Allergens: Dogs with food allergies or sensitivities may react to certain ingredients commonly found in commercial dog food, such as grains, artificial preservatives, or meat by-

products.

3. Processing Methods: The processing methods used in commercial dog food production, such as high-heat cooking or extrusion, can degrade the nutritional value of ingredients and reduce the bioavailability of nutrients.

4. Limited Variety: While commercial dog foods offer a range of options, including different flavors and formulations, they may lack the variety and freshness of homemade meals. Dogs may become bored with the same commercial diet over time.

Ultimately, the decision between homemade and commercial dog food depends on your dog's individual needs, your lifestyle, and your comfort level with meal preparation. Whether you choose to feed homemade or commercial food, prioritizing balanced nutrition and consulting with a veterinarian or veterinary nutritionist will ensure your dog receives the best care possible.

Pros of Homemade Dog Food:

1. Control Over Ingredients: You have complete control over the quality and source of ingredients, allowing you to tailor the diet to your dog's specific nutritional needs and preferences.

2. Freshness and Quality: Homemade dog food often uses fresh, whole ingredients without artificial preservatives or additives, promoting better overall health and well-being.

3. Customization for Dietary Restrictions: Homemade diets are ideal for dogs with food allergies, sensitivities, or specific dietary restrictions, as you can easily avoid common allergens and customize the diet accordingly.

4. Bonding Experience: Cooking for your dog can strengthen the bond between you and your furry friend, providing a rewarding experience and an opportunity to show love and care through homemade meals.

Cons of Homemade Dog Food:

1. Time-Consuming: Preparing homemade dog food requires significant time and effort, including meal planning, shopping for ingredients, and cooking, which can be challenging for busy pet

parents.

2. Nutritional Imbalance: Without proper knowledge and guidance, homemade dog food may be nutritionally imbalanced, leading to deficiencies or excesses of essential nutrients. It's essential to consult with a veterinarian or veterinary nutritionist to ensure the diet meets your dog's needs.

3. Cost: Homemade dog food can be more expensive than commercial options, especially if you're using high-quality, organic ingredients. The cost of ingredients, supplements, and kitchen equipment adds up over time.

4. Potential for Contamination: Improper handling or storage of homemade dog food can increase the risk of bacterial contamination, leading to foodborne illnesses in dogs. It's crucial to follow proper food safety practices to minimize this risk.

Overall, homemade dog food offers benefits such as ingredient control, freshness, customization, and bonding opportunities, but it requires time, knowledge, and careful planning to ensure it meets your dog's nutritional needs effectively. Consulting with a veterinarian or veterinary nutritionist can provide valuable guidance and support in creating a balanced homemade diet for your canine companion.

Understanding Commercial Dog Food Labels

Deciphering commercial dog food labels can be challenging, but it's essential for ensuring you're making informed decisions about your dog's diet. Here's a guide to understanding the key components of commercial dog food labels:

1. Ingredient List:

   - Ingredients are listed in descending order by weight, with the heaviest ingredients listed first.

   - Look for named protein sources (e.g., chicken, beef, lamb) as the first few ingredients, indicating a higher quality protein content.

   - Avoid foods with generic meat by-products or vague ingredient descriptions, as they may contain lower quality or unspecified protein sources.

2. Guaranteed Analysis:
- Provides minimum and maximum percentages of crude protein, crude fat, crude fiber, and moisture in the food.
- Use these percentages as a rough guide to assess the overall nutrient content of the food, but keep in mind that they may not reflect the actual digestibility or bioavailability of nutrients.

3. Nutritional Adequacy Statement:
- Indicates whether the food is formulated to meet the nutritional levels established by the Association of American Feed Control Officials (AAFCO) for a specific life stage (e.g., adult maintenance, growth, or all life stages).
- Look for statements such as "complete and balanced" or "formulated to meet the nutritional levels established by AAFCO" to ensure the food is nutritionally adequate for your dog's needs.

4. Feeding Guidelines:
- Provides recommended feeding amounts based on your dog's weight and/or age.
- Follow these guidelines closely to prevent overfeeding or underfeeding your dog, adjusting portion sizes as needed based on your dog's activity level, metabolism, and body condition.

5. Additional Information:
- Look for additional information such as feeding instructions, storage recommendations, expiration date, and contact information for the manufacturer.
- Pay attention to any special claims or certifications (e.g., organic, grain-free, limited ingredient) and consider whether they align with your dog's dietary preferences or health needs.

6. Understanding Additives and Preservatives:
- Be cautious of artificial additives and preservatives such as BHA, BHT, ethoxyquin, and artificial colors or flavors, which may be harmful to your dog's health.
- Opt for foods with natural preservatives such as tocopherols

(vitamin E) or rosemary extract, or choose preservative-free options if available.

By understanding and interpreting commercial dog food labels, you can make more informed choices about the foods you're feeding your furry friend, ensuring they receive a balanced and nutritious diet tailored to their individual needs. If you have any questions or concerns about specific ingredients or nutritional requirements, don't hesitate to consult with a veterinarian or veterinary nutritionist for personalized guidance.

Transitioning your dog to homemade food safely requires careful planning and gradual changes to prevent digestive upset or nutritional imbalances. Here's a step-by-step guide to help you transition your dog to homemade food:

1. Consult with a Veterinarian or Veterinary Nutritionist:
   - Before making any dietary changes, consult with a veterinarian or veterinary nutritionist to ensure homemade food is appropriate for your dog's age, breed, health status, and nutritional needs.
   - They can provide personalized guidance, recommend appropriate recipes, and help you formulate a balanced diet that meets your dog's requirements.

2. Research and Recipe Selection:
   - Research homemade dog food recipes from reputable sources such as veterinary nutritionists, certified canine nutritionists, or trusted pet food websites.
   - Choose recipes that are balanced, nutritionally complete, and tailored to your dog's specific needs, considering factors such as age, weight, activity level, and any dietary restrictions or allergies.

3. Gradual Transition:
   - Start by mixing a small amount of homemade food with your dog's current commercial diet, gradually increasing the proportion of homemade food over time.
   - Aim to transition your dog to homemade food over the course

of 7-10 days, adjusting the ratio of homemade to commercial food gradually to allow your dog's digestive system to adapt.

4. Monitor Your Dog's Response:
- Monitor your dog closely during the transition period for any signs of digestive upset, such as diarrhea, vomiting, or changes in appetite or energy levels.
- If your dog experiences digestive issues, slow down the transition process, revert to the previous diet, or consult with your veterinarian for guidance.

5. Ensure Balanced Nutrition:
- Ensure that the homemade diet provides a balanced and complete nutrition profile, including adequate levels of protein, carbohydrates, fats, vitamins, and minerals.
- Use a variety of ingredients to ensure nutritional variety and prevent deficiencies. Include sources of lean protein, healthy fats, whole grains, and fruits and vegetables in your dog's diet.

6. Supplement as Needed:
- Consider supplementing your dog's homemade diet with additional nutrients or supplements if recommended by your veterinarian or veterinary nutritionist.
- Common supplements for homemade dog food may include omega-3 fatty acids (e.g., fish oil), calcium, vitamin D, or multivitamin/mineral supplements.

7. Regular Monitoring and Adjustments:
- Monitor your dog's body condition, energy levels, and overall health regularly after transitioning to homemade food.
- Be prepared to make adjustments to the diet as needed based on your dog's response, activity level, and any changes in health status.

By following these steps and working closely with your veterinarian or veterinary nutritionist, you can safely transition your dog to a homemade diet that meets their nutritional needs and promotes their overall health and well-being.

Chapter 3: Kitchen Essentials For Homemade Dog Food

Embarking on the journey of preparing homemade dog food requires the right tools and equipment to ensure safe and efficient meal preparation. In this chapter, we'll explore the essential kitchen essentials for creating nutritious and delicious homemade meals for your canine companion.

1. Stainless Steel Bowls:
   - Durable and easy to clean, stainless steel bowls are ideal for mixing and serving homemade dog food.
   - Choose bowls of appropriate size for your dog's portion sizes and meal frequency.

2. Cutting Board and Sharp Knives:
   - A sturdy cutting board and sharp knives are essential for chopping and preparing ingredients such as meats, vegetables, and fruits.
   - Opt for a cutting board made of non-porous material, such as plastic or wood, to prevent cross-contamination.

3. Food Processor or Blender:
   - A food processor or blender is useful for pureeing ingredients, especially for dogs with dental issues or smaller breeds that may have difficulty chewing.
   - Use a food processor to finely chop vegetables, fruits, or meats, or to create smooth textures for homemade dog food recipes.

4. Cooking Utensils:
   - Stock your kitchen with essential cooking utensils such as spatulas, ladles, stirring spoons, and measuring cups and spoons.
   - These utensils will help you accurately portion ingredients, mix recipes, and transfer food safely during the cooking process.

5. Pots and Pans:

- Invest in a variety of pots and pans of different sizes for cooking and simmering homemade dog food recipes.
- Choose pots and pans made of stainless steel or non-stick materials for easy cleaning and durability.

6. Storage Containers:
- Proper storage containers are essential for storing homemade dog food safely in the refrigerator or freezer.
- Use airtight containers made of glass or BPA-free plastic to keep homemade meals fresh and prevent contamination.

7. Kitchen Scale:
- A kitchen scale is invaluable for accurately measuring ingredients and portion sizes when preparing homemade dog food recipes.
- Use a digital kitchen scale to measure ingredients by weight, ensuring consistency and precision in your recipes.

8. Food Safety Essentials:
- Practice proper food safety techniques when preparing homemade dog food, including washing hands, surfaces, and utensils thoroughly before and after handling raw ingredients.
- Use separate cutting boards and utensils for preparing dog food to prevent cross-contamination with human food.

9. Blender for bone grinding:
- A blender with a strong motor is essential for grinding bones if your homemade dog food recipe includes bone-in meats.
- Use a blender with sharp blades and a powerful motor to grind bones to a safe and appropriate consistency for your dog's consumption.

10. Food Storage Bags:
- Keep food storage bags on hand for portioning and storing homemade dog food in individual servings or for long-term freezer storage.
- Choose freezer-safe bags with secure seals to maintain freshness and prevent freezer burn.

By equipping your kitchen with these essential tools and equipment, you'll be well-prepared to prepare nutritious and delicious homemade meals for your beloved canine companion. Remember to prioritize food safety and proper handling practices to ensure the health and well-being of your dog.

Essential Tools and Equipment for Homemade Dog Food Preparation:

1. **Stainless Steel Bowls**: Durable and easy to clean, stainless steel bowls are ideal for mixing and serving homemade dog food.

2. **Cutting Board and Sharp Knives**: A sturdy cutting board and sharp knives are essential for chopping and preparing ingredients such as meats, vegetables, and fruits.

3. **Food Processor or Blender**: Useful for pureeing ingredients and creating smooth textures, especially for dogs with dental issues or smaller breeds.

4. **Cooking Utensils**: Spatulas, ladles, stirring spoons, and measuring cups and spoons help accurately portion ingredients and mix recipes.

5. **Pots and Pans**: Various sizes of pots and pans are needed for cooking and simmering homemade dog food recipes.

6. **Storage Containers**: Airtight containers made of glass or BPA-free plastic are necessary for storing homemade meals safely in the refrigerator or freezer.

7. **Kitchen Scale**: For accurately measuring ingredients and portion sizes, ensuring consistency and precision in recipes.

8. **Blender for Bone Grinding**: Essential if your recipe includes bone-in meats, a powerful blender can grind bones to a safe consistency for consumption.

9. **Food Storage Bags**: Useful for portioning and storing homemade dog food in individual servings or for long-term

freezer storage.

10. **Food Safety Essentials**: Wash hands, surfaces, and utensils thoroughly before and after handling raw ingredients, and use separate tools for preparing dog food to prevent cross-contamination.

With these essential tools and equipment, you'll be well-equipped to prepare nutritious and delicious homemade meals for your furry friend.
Safe food handling practices are essential when preparing homemade dog food to ensure the health and well-being of your canine companion. Here are some key practices to follow:

1. **Cleanliness**: Wash your hands thoroughly with soap and water before and after handling raw ingredients, as well as any surfaces, utensils, and equipment used in food preparation.

2. **Separation**: Use separate cutting boards, utensils, and kitchen equipment for preparing dog food to prevent cross-contamination with human food.

3. **Fresh Ingredients**: Use fresh, high-quality ingredients and check for any signs of spoilage or contamination before using them in recipes.

4. **Cooking Temperatures**: Cook meats, grains, and other ingredients to appropriate temperatures to kill harmful bacteria and pathogens. Use a food thermometer to ensure food reaches the recommended safe internal temperature.

5. **Storage**: Store homemade dog food in airtight containers in the refrigerator or freezer to maintain freshness and prevent bacterial growth. Label containers with the date of preparation and use within a reasonable timeframe.

6. **Thawing**: Thaw frozen homemade dog food in the refrigerator or microwave, never at room temperature, to prevent bacterial growth.

7. **Portioning**: Portion homemade dog food into individual servings to minimize the risk of contamination during feeding. Use clean utensils and wash food bowls regularly with hot, soapy water.

8. **Monitoring**: Monitor your dog's reaction to homemade food for any signs of digestive upset, such as diarrhea, vomiting, or changes in appetite or energy levels. Consult with a veterinarian if you notice any adverse reactions.

9. **Hydration**: Ensure your dog has access to fresh, clean water at all times, especially when feeding dry or homemade food, to prevent dehydration.

10. **Consultation**: Consult with a veterinarian or veterinary nutritionist before making any significant changes to your dog's diet, especially if they have underlying health conditions or special dietary needs.

By following these safe food handling practices, you can minimize the risk of foodborne illness and ensure that your homemade dog food is safe, nutritious, and beneficial for your furry friend's health and well-being.
Storing homemade dog food properly is essential to maintain its freshness, nutritional integrity, and safety. Here are some tips for storing homemade dog food:

1. **Airtight Containers**: Use airtight containers made of glass, BPA-free plastic, or stainless steel to store homemade dog food. This helps prevent exposure to air, moisture, and contaminants, preserving freshness and flavor.

2. **Refrigeration**: Store homemade dog food in the refrigerator if you plan to use it within a few days. Divide the food into smaller portions and store them in individual containers for easy serving. Label containers with the date of preparation for reference.

3. **Freezing**: If you're preparing large batches of homemade

dog food or want to store it for an extended period, freezing is the best option. Portion the food into freezer-safe containers or resealable bags, removing excess air to prevent freezer burn. Label containers with the date of preparation and contents for easy identification.

4. **Thawing**: Thaw frozen homemade dog food in the refrigerator overnight or in the microwave using the defrost setting. Avoid thawing at room temperature, as this can promote bacterial growth.

5. **Use within Recommended Timeframe**: Homemade dog food stored in the refrigerator should be used within 3-5 days to maintain freshness and safety. Frozen homemade dog food can be stored for up to 2-3 months for optimal quality.

6. **Rotate Stock**: If you regularly prepare homemade dog food, rotate your stock by using older batches first to prevent food waste and ensure freshness.

7. **Avoid Overfilling**: Fill containers with homemade dog food leaving some space at the top to allow for expansion during freezing and to prevent leaks.

8. **Inspect for Spoilage**: Before serving homemade dog food, inspect it for any signs of spoilage, such as mold, off-odor, or unusual discoloration. Discard any food that appears spoiled or questionable.

9. **Maintain Hygiene**: Wash your hands, utensils, and storage containers thoroughly before and after handling homemade dog food to prevent contamination.

10. **Consult with a Veterinarian**: If you have any concerns about storing homemade dog food or if your dog has specific dietary needs or health conditions, consult with a veterinarian or veterinary nutritionist for personalized guidance and recommendations.

By following these tips for storing homemade dog food, you can ensure that it remains fresh, safe, and nutritious for your canine companion's enjoyment and well-being.

Chapter 4: Building Balanced Meals For Dogs

Creating balanced meals for your dog is essential to ensure they receive the nutrients they need for optimal health and well-being. In this chapter, we'll explore the key components of balanced meals for dogs and how to tailor their diet to meet their specific nutritional needs.

Understanding Nutritional Needs:
- Dogs require a balanced diet that includes proteins, carbohydrates, fats, vitamins, and minerals to support their growth, energy, and overall health.
- The amount and type of nutrients your dog needs depend on factors such as age, breed, size, activity level, and any underlying health conditions.

Key Components of Balanced Meals:
1. Protein:
   - Protein is crucial for building and repairing tissues, muscles, and cells in your dog's body.
   - High-quality protein sources include meat, poultry, fish, eggs, and plant-based sources such as legumes and tofu.

2. Carbohydrates:
   - Carbohydrates provide energy and fiber for your dog's daily activities and digestive health.
   - Choose complex carbohydrates such as whole grains (e.g., brown rice, oats, quinoa), vegetables (e.g., sweet potatoes, carrots, broccoli), and fruits (e.g., apples, berries) for added nutrients and fiber.

3. Fats:
   - Fats are a concentrated source of energy and essential fatty acids (omega-3 and omega-6) that support your dog's skin, coat, and immune system.
   - Include healthy fats from sources such as fish oil, flaxseed oil,

coconut oil, and animal fats in moderation.

4. Vitamins and Minerals:
   - Vitamins and minerals play vital roles in various bodily functions, including immune support, bone health, and metabolism.
   - Ensure your dog's diet includes a balanced variety of vitamins and minerals from sources such as fruits, vegetables, whole grains, and supplements if necessary.

5. Water:
   - Water is essential for your dog's hydration, digestion, and overall health.
   - Provide fresh, clean water at all times, especially during and after meals, and monitor your dog's water intake to prevent dehydration.

Meal Planning and Portion Control:
- Create a meal plan that includes a balance of proteins, carbohydrates, and fats, tailored to your dog's specific needs and preferences.
- Divide your dog's daily food intake into multiple meals throughout the day to promote digestion and prevent overeating.
- Monitor your dog's body condition and adjust portion sizes as needed to maintain a healthy weight and body condition score.

By building balanced meals that incorporate a variety of high-quality ingredients, you can ensure your dog receives the nutrients they need to thrive. Consulting with a veterinarian or veterinary nutritionist can provide personalized guidance and recommendations for creating a balanced diet that meets your dog's individual needs.

Each nutrient plays a crucial role in supporting your dog's overall health and well-being. Here's a breakdown of the roles of protein, carbohydrates, fats, vitamins, and minerals in your dog's diet:

1. Protein:
   - Role: Protein is essential for building and repairing tissues,

muscles, and cells in your dog's body. It provides the necessary amino acids for various physiological functions.

- Sources: High-quality protein sources for dogs include meat, poultry, fish, eggs, and plant-based sources such as legumes and tofu.

- Importance: Adequate protein intake is crucial for growth and development, maintaining muscle mass, supporting immune function, and overall health.

2. Carbohydrates:

- Role: Carbohydrates are the primary source of energy for your dog's body, providing fuel for daily activities and metabolic processes. They also contribute fiber for digestive health.

- Sources: Complex carbohydrates such as whole grains (e.g., brown rice, oats, quinoa), vegetables (e.g., sweet potatoes, carrots, broccoli), and fruits (e.g., apples, berries) are ideal choices.

- Importance: Carbohydrates support energy metabolism, regulate blood sugar levels, promote satiety, and provide essential nutrients and fiber for digestive health.

3. Fats:

- Role: Fats serve as a concentrated source of energy and are essential for the absorption of fat-soluble vitamins (A, D, E, and K). They also provide essential fatty acids (omega-3 and omega-6) that support skin, coat, and immune function.

- Sources: Healthy fat sources for dogs include fish oil, flaxseed oil, coconut oil, and animal fats from meats.

- Importance: Fats play a critical role in maintaining healthy skin and coat, supporting brain function, regulating inflammation, and providing essential nutrients and energy for overall health.

4. Vitamins:

- Role: Vitamins are organic compounds that play various roles in metabolism, growth, and immune function. They act as coenzymes and antioxidants, supporting cellular processes and protecting against oxidative damage.

- Sources: Vitamins are found in a variety of foods, including fruits, vegetables, meats, grains, and supplements.

- Importance: Vitamins are essential for maintaining overall health, supporting immune function, promoting growth and development, and preventing deficiencies and diseases.

5. Minerals:

- Role: Minerals are inorganic nutrients that play critical roles in bone and teeth formation, muscle function, fluid balance, and enzyme activity. They are essential for various physiological processes in the body.

- Sources: Minerals are found in a wide range of foods, including meats, grains, fruits, vegetables, and supplements.

- Importance: Minerals are essential for maintaining structural integrity, regulating cellular processes, supporting growth and development, and preventing deficiencies and diseases.

By providing a balanced diet that includes adequate amounts of protein, carbohydrates, fats, vitamins, and minerals, you can support your dog's overall health, growth, and vitality. Consulting with a veterinarian or veterinary nutritionist can help ensure your dog's nutritional needs are met and address any specific dietary requirements or concerns.

Recommended nutrient ratios for different life stages and breeds can vary based on factors such as age, size, activity level, and health status. However, here are some general guidelines for recommended nutrient ratios:

1. **Puppies**:
   - Protein: 22-32% of total calories
   - Fat: 8-12% of total calories
   - Carbohydrates: 45-55% of total calories
   - Calcium: 1.0-1.8%
   - Phosphorus: 0.8-1.6%
   - Energy Density: Higher to support growth and development

2. **Adult Dogs**:

- Protein: 18-25% of total calories
- Fat: 5-15% of total calories
- Carbohydrates: 30-70% of total calories (varies based on activity level and metabolism)
- Calcium: 0.5-1.3%
- Phosphorus: 0.4-1.0%
- Energy Density: Moderate to maintain ideal body condition

3. **Senior Dogs**:
   - Protein: 18-25% of total calories
   - Fat: 5-12% of total calories
   - Carbohydrates: 30-60% of total calories (varies based on activity level and metabolism)
   - Calcium: 0.5-1.0%
   - Phosphorus: 0.3-0.8%
   - Energy Density: Lower to prevent obesity and support aging metabolism

4. **Large Breed Dogs**:
   - Protein: 20-25% of total calories
   - Fat: 10-15% of total calories
   - Carbohydrates: 45-55% of total calories
   - Calcium: 0.7-1.0%
   - Phosphorus: 0.5-0.8%
   - Energy Density: Moderate to support growth without excessive weight gain

5. **Small Breed Dogs**:
   - Protein: 20-30% of total calories
   - Fat: 10-20% of total calories
   - Carbohydrates: 30-60% of total calories
   - Calcium: 0.8-1.3%
   - Phosphorus: 0.6-1.0%
   - Energy Density: Higher to meet energy needs in smaller portions

It's essential to consider your dog's individual needs,

preferences, and any underlying health conditions when determining the ideal nutrient ratios for their diet. Consulting with a veterinarian or veterinary nutritionist can provide personalized recommendations and ensure your dog's nutritional requirements are met throughout their life stages.

Choosing the best ingredients for your dog's needs involves considering factors such as their age, size, activity level, dietary preferences, and any underlying health conditions. Here are some tips for selecting ingredients to meet your dog's nutritional requirements:

1. **High-Quality Protein Sources**:
   - Choose lean, high-quality protein sources such as chicken, turkey, beef, fish, eggs, and plant-based sources like lentils or chickpeas.
   - Consider your dog's protein requirements based on factors such as age, size, activity level, and any dietary restrictions or allergies.

2. **Healthy Fats**:
   - Include healthy fats from sources such as fish oil, flaxseed oil, coconut oil, and animal fats to support skin, coat, and overall health.
   - Ensure a balanced ratio of omega-3 and omega-6 fatty acids for optimal health benefits.

3. **Complex Carbohydrates**:
   - Choose complex carbohydrates such as brown rice, oats, quinoa, sweet potatoes, and vegetables like carrots, broccoli, and spinach.
   - Avoid refined grains and high-glycemic carbohydrates that can cause spikes in blood sugar levels.

4. **Fruits and Vegetables**:
   - Incorporate a variety of fruits and vegetables into your dog's diet to provide essential vitamins, minerals, and antioxidants.
   - Include colorful fruits and vegetables like blueberries, apples,

pumpkin, and leafy greens for added nutritional benefits.

5. **Supplements**:
   - Consider adding supplements such as fish oil for omega-3 fatty acids, glucosamine and chondroitin for joint health, and probiotics for digestive health, as recommended by your veterinarian.
   - Choose supplements from reputable brands and consult with your veterinarian for proper dosage and administration.

6. **Avoid Harmful Ingredients**:
   - Avoid ingredients that can be harmful to dogs, such as onions, garlic, grapes, raisins, chocolate, caffeine, xylitol, and artificial sweeteners.
   - Read ingredient labels carefully and avoid foods with artificial preservatives, colors, and fillers.

7. **Tailor to Dietary Restrictions**:
   - If your dog has food allergies, sensitivities, or specific dietary restrictions, choose ingredients that are suitable for their needs.
   - Consult with your veterinarian or veterinary nutritionist for guidance on selecting appropriate ingredients and formulating a balanced diet.

8. **Variety and Balance**:
   - Provide a balanced diet that includes a variety of ingredients to ensure your dog receives all the essential nutrients they need.
   - Rotate protein sources, carbohydrates, fruits, and vegetables to prevent nutrient deficiencies and boredom with their diet.

By carefully selecting high-quality ingredients that meet your dog's nutritional needs and preferences, you can ensure they enjoy a balanced and nutritious diet that supports their overall health and well-being. Consulting with a veterinarian or veterinary nutritionist can provide personalized recommendations and guidance for selecting the best ingredients for your dog's specific needs.

Chapter 5: Meaty Marvels: Protein-Packed Recipes

In this chapter, we'll explore a variety of protein-packed recipes that will delight your dog's taste buds and provide them with the essential nutrients they need to thrive. These homemade recipes feature high-quality protein sources and wholesome ingredients to support your dog's health and well-being.

1. **Chicken and Sweet Potato Stew**:
   - Ingredients: Boneless chicken breast or thighs, sweet potatoes, carrots, peas, chicken broth (low sodium), olive oil.
   - Method: Cook the chicken until fully cooked, then shred. In a pot, simmer sweet potatoes, carrots, and peas in chicken broth until tender. Add shredded chicken and a drizzle of olive oil. Serve once cooled.

2. **Beef and Brown Rice Casserole**:
   - Ingredients: Lean ground beef, brown rice, spinach, carrots, beef broth (low sodium), olive oil.
   - Method: Brown the ground beef in a skillet until cooked through. Cook brown rice according to package instructions. In a casserole dish, layer cooked beef, rice, chopped spinach, and carrots. Pour beef broth over the mixture and bake until vegetables are tender.

3. **Salmon and Quinoa Salad**:
   - Ingredients: Canned salmon (in water), cooked quinoa, green beans, bell peppers, olive oil, lemon juice.
   - Method: Drain canned salmon and flake into a bowl. Add cooked quinoa, blanched green beans, diced bell peppers, a drizzle of olive oil, and a squeeze of lemon juice. Mix well and serve chilled.

4. **Turkey and Pumpkin Meatballs**:
   - Ingredients: Ground turkey, canned pumpkin puree, oats, eggs, parsley, olive oil.

- Method: Mix ground turkey, pumpkin puree, oats, beaten eggs, and chopped parsley in a bowl until well combined. Form into meatballs and place on a baking sheet. Drizzle with olive oil and bake until cooked through.

5. **Lamb and Lentil Stew**:
   - Ingredients: Ground lamb, lentils, carrots, celery, tomatoes (diced), beef broth (low sodium), garlic powder, rosemary.
   - Method: Brown ground lamb in a pot, then add lentils, chopped carrots, celery, diced tomatoes, and beef broth. Season with garlic powder and rosemary. Simmer until lentils are tender and flavors are well combined.

These protein-packed recipes offer a delicious and nutritious alternative to commercial dog food, providing your canine companion with the essential nutrients they need to thrive. Feel free to customize the ingredients and adjust portion sizes based on your dog's preferences and dietary needs. Always consult with your veterinarian before introducing new foods or making significant changes to your dog's diet.

Chicken and Sweet Potato Stew Recipe:

Ingredients:
- 2 boneless, skinless chicken breasts
- 2 sweet potatoes, peeled and diced
- 1 cup carrots, chopped
- 1/2 cup frozen peas
- 2 cups chicken broth (low sodium)
- 1 tablespoon olive oil

Instructions:
1. In a large pot, heat olive oil over medium heat. Add the chicken breasts and cook until browned on both sides, about 5-7 minutes per side. Remove chicken from the pot and set aside.
2. In the same pot, add the diced sweet potatoes and carrots. Cook for 5 minutes, stirring occasionally.
3. Pour in the chicken broth and bring to a boil. Reduce heat to low

and simmer for 10-15 minutes, or until the vegetables are tender.
4. While the vegetables are cooking, shred the cooked chicken breasts using two forks.
5. Once the vegetables are tender, add the shredded chicken and frozen peas to the pot. Stir to combine.
6. Simmer for an additional 5 minutes, or until the peas are heated through.
7. Remove from heat and let cool before serving to your dog. Store any leftovers in an airtight container in the refrigerator for up to 3 days.

This Chicken and Sweet Potato Stew is packed with protein, vitamins, and minerals, making it a nutritious and delicious meal option for your furry friend. Adjust the portion sizes and ingredients based on your dog's size and dietary needs. Always consult with your veterinarian before introducing new foods or making significant changes to your dog's diet.
Beef and Barley Casserole Recipe:

Ingredients:
- 1 lb lean ground beef
- 1 cup barley, rinsed
- 2 cups beef broth (low sodium)
- 1 cup diced carrots
- 1 cup diced celery
- 1 cup diced bell peppers (any color)
- 1 tablespoon olive oil
- 1 teaspoon dried thyme
- Salt and pepper to taste

Instructions:
1. Preheat your oven to 375°F (190°C). Lightly grease a casserole dish with olive oil.
2. In a large skillet, heat olive oil over medium heat. Add the ground beef and cook until browned, breaking it into crumbles with a spatula.
3. Add the diced carrots, celery, and bell peppers to the skillet.

Cook for 5 minutes, until the vegetables start to soften.
4. Stir in the rinsed barley and dried thyme. Cook for another 2 minutes, allowing the barley to toast slightly.
5. Transfer the beef and vegetable mixture to the greased casserole dish. Spread it out evenly.
6. Pour the beef broth over the mixture in the casserole dish. Stir gently to combine.
7. Cover the casserole dish with aluminum foil and bake in the preheated oven for 45-50 minutes, or until the barley is tender and most of the liquid is absorbed.
8. Remove the foil and bake for an additional 10 minutes to allow the top to brown slightly.
9. Let the casserole cool for a few minutes before serving to your dog. Store any leftovers in an airtight container in the refrigerator for up to 3 days.

This Beef and Barley Casserole is hearty, nutritious, and packed with protein and fiber, making it a satisfying meal for your furry friend. Adjust the ingredients and portion sizes based on your dog's size and dietary needs. Always consult with your veterinarian before introducing new foods or making significant changes to your dog's diet.

Turkey and Vegetable Stir-Fry Recipe:

Ingredients:
- 1 lb ground turkey
- 2 cups mixed vegetables (such as bell peppers, broccoli, carrots, snap peas)
- 2 cloves garlic, minced
- 1 tablespoon ginger, minced
- 2 tablespoons low-sodium soy sauce or tamari
- 1 tablespoon olive oil
- Cooked brown rice or quinoa for serving

Instructions:
1. Heat olive oil in a large skillet or wok over medium-high heat.
2. Add minced garlic and ginger to the skillet and cook for 1

minute until fragrant.

3. Add ground turkey to the skillet and cook until browned, breaking it into crumbles with a spatula.

4. Add mixed vegetables to the skillet and cook for 3-4 minutes, until they start to soften but are still crisp.

5. Stir in low-sodium soy sauce or tamari, ensuring all ingredients are well coated.

6. Continue to cook for another 2-3 minutes, stirring occasionally, until the vegetables are tender and the turkey is fully cooked.

7. Remove from heat and let cool slightly before serving.

8. Serve the turkey and vegetable stir-fry over cooked brown rice or quinoa.

9. Allow the stir-fry to cool completely before serving to your dog.

10. Store any leftovers in an airtight container in the refrigerator for up to 3 days.

This Turkey and Vegetable Stir-Fry is a delicious and nutritious meal option for your furry friend, packed with lean protein and a variety of colorful vegetables. Adjust the ingredients and seasonings based on your dog's preferences and dietary needs. Always consult with your veterinarian before introducing new foods or making significant changes to your dog's diet.

Chapter 6: Carb Creations: Wholesome Grain And Vegetable Dishes

In this chapter, we'll explore a collection of nutritious and delicious grain and vegetable dishes that will delight your dog's palate while providing essential carbohydrates, fiber, vitamins, and minerals. These homemade recipes feature wholesome ingredients and are easy to prepare, making them perfect for incorporating into your dog's diet.

1. **Brown Rice and Vegetable Medley**:
   - Ingredients: Cooked brown rice, mixed vegetables (such as carrots, peas, green beans), olive oil.
   - Method: Mix cooked brown rice with steamed or lightly sautéed mixed vegetables. Drizzle with a small amount of olive oil for added flavor and healthy fats. Serve as a standalone dish or mix with lean protein for a balanced meal.

2. **Quinoa and Spinach Salad**:
   - Ingredients: Cooked quinoa, fresh spinach leaves, cherry tomatoes, cucumber, olive oil, lemon juice.
   - Method: Toss cooked quinoa with fresh spinach leaves, halved cherry tomatoes, and diced cucumber. Dress with a mixture of olive oil and lemon juice for a refreshing and nutritious salad.

3. **Sweet Potato and Lentil Stew**:
   - Ingredients: Cooked lentils, mashed sweet potatoes, carrots, celery, vegetable broth, parsley.
   - Method: Combine cooked lentils with mashed sweet potatoes and diced carrots and celery. Add vegetable broth to achieve desired consistency and simmer until vegetables are tender. Garnish with chopped parsley before serving.

4. **Pumpkin and Oatmeal Cookies**:
   - Ingredients: Canned pumpkin puree, rolled oats, banana, cinnamon, honey (optional).

- Method: Mash ripe banana and mix with canned pumpkin puree, rolled oats, and a dash of cinnamon. Form mixture into small cookies and place on a baking sheet. Bake at a low temperature until firm and golden brown. Allow to cool before serving.

5. **Barley and Vegetable Risotto**:
   - Ingredients: Cooked barley, mixed vegetables (such as mushrooms, bell peppers, zucchini), low-sodium vegetable broth, grated Parmesan cheese (optional).
   - Method: Sauté mixed vegetables in a skillet until tender. Stir in cooked barley and gradually add vegetable broth, stirring frequently, until creamy and well combined. Serve with a sprinkle of grated Parmesan cheese if desired.

These carb creations offer a variety of nutrient-rich options to complement your dog's diet and provide them with essential carbohydrates, fiber, and vitamins. Feel free to customize the ingredients and adjust portion sizes based on your dog's preferences and dietary needs. Always consult with your veterinarian before introducing new foods or making significant changes to your dog's diet.
Brown Rice and Lentil Medley Recipe:

Ingredients:
- 1 cup brown rice
- 1/2 cup dried green or brown lentils
- 2 cups water or low-sodium vegetable broth
- 1 tablespoon olive oil
- 1 carrot, diced
- 1 stalk celery, diced
- 1/2 cup frozen peas
- 1/2 teaspoon dried thyme (optional)
- Salt and pepper to taste

Instructions:
1. Rinse the brown rice and lentils under cold water.

2. In a medium saucepan, heat olive oil over medium heat. Add diced carrot and celery, and sauté for 3-4 minutes until slightly softened.
3. Add brown rice, lentils, water or vegetable broth, and dried thyme to the saucepan. Bring to a boil.
4. Once boiling, reduce heat to low, cover, and simmer for 35-40 minutes, or until the rice and lentils are tender and the liquid is absorbed.
5. Stir in the frozen peas during the last 5 minutes of cooking.
6. Remove from heat and let the medley cool before serving to your dog.
7. Season with salt and pepper to taste.
8. Serve as a standalone dish or mix with lean protein for a balanced meal.
9. Store any leftovers in an airtight container in the refrigerator for up to 3 days.

This Brown Rice and Lentil Medley is a nutritious and filling dish for your furry friend, packed with fiber, protein, and essential nutrients. Adjust the ingredients and portion sizes based on your dog's size and dietary needs. Always consult with your veterinarian before introducing new foods or making significant changes to your dog's diet.

Quinoa and Spinach Delight Recipe:

Ingredients:
- 1 cup quinoa, rinsed
- 2 cups low-sodium vegetable broth or water
- 2 cups fresh spinach leaves, chopped
- 1/2 cup cherry tomatoes, halved
- 1/2 cup cucumber, diced
- 1 tablespoon olive oil
- 1 tablespoon lemon juice
- Salt and pepper to taste

Instructions:
1. In a medium saucepan, combine quinoa and vegetable broth or

water. Bring to a boil.

2. Reduce heat to low, cover, and simmer for 15-20 minutes, or until the quinoa is cooked and the liquid is absorbed.

3. In a large mixing bowl, combine cooked quinoa, chopped spinach leaves, halved cherry tomatoes, and diced cucumber.

4. In a small bowl, whisk together olive oil and lemon juice to make the dressing.

5. Pour the dressing over the quinoa and vegetable mixture. Toss to coat evenly.

6. Season with salt and pepper to taste.

7. Let the quinoa and spinach delight cool before serving to your dog.

8. Serve as a standalone dish or mix with lean protein for a balanced meal.

9. Store any leftovers in an airtight container in the refrigerator for up to 3 days.

This Quinoa and Spinach Delight is a refreshing and nutritious dish for your furry friend, packed with protein, fiber, vitamins, and minerals. Adjust the ingredients and portion sizes based on your dog's size and dietary needs. Always consult with your veterinarian before introducing new foods or making significant changes to your dog's diet.

Pumpkin and Oatmeal Bake Recipe:

Ingredients:

- 1 cup canned pumpkin puree (make sure it's 100% pumpkin, not pumpkin pie filling)
- 1 cup rolled oats (not instant oats)
- 1 ripe banana, mashed
- 1 teaspoon ground cinnamon
- 1 tablespoon honey (optional)
- Coconut oil or cooking spray for greasing the baking dish

Instructions:

1. Preheat your oven to 350°F (175°C). Grease a small baking dish with coconut oil or cooking spray.

2. In a mixing bowl, combine the canned pumpkin puree, rolled oats, mashed banana, ground cinnamon, and honey (if using). Mix until well combined.

3. Transfer the mixture to the greased baking dish, spreading it out evenly.

4. Bake in the preheated oven for 25-30 minutes, or until the edges are golden brown and the bake is set in the center.

5. Remove from the oven and let it cool completely before cutting into squares or bars.

6. Serve the pumpkin and oatmeal bake as a tasty and nutritious treat for your dog.

7. Store any leftovers in an airtight container in the refrigerator for up to 3 days.

This Pumpkin and Oatmeal Bake is a wholesome and satisfying treat for your furry friend, packed with fiber, vitamins, and minerals. Adjust the ingredients and portion sizes based on your dog's size and dietary needs. Always consult with your veterinarian before introducing new foods or treats into your dog's diet.

Chapter 7: Healthy Treats And Snacks For Happy Pups

In this chapter, we'll explore a variety of wholesome and nutritious treats and snacks that will keep your pup happy and healthy. These homemade recipes are easy to make and use simple, natural ingredients to provide your dog with tasty rewards and snacks.

1. **Peanut Butter and Banana Bites**:
   - Ingredients: Ripe bananas, natural peanut butter (make sure it doesn't contain xylitol), rolled oats.
   - Method: Mash ripe bananas and mix with natural peanut butter and rolled oats. Form into bite-sized balls and refrigerate until firm. Serve as a tasty and protein-packed treat.

2. **Carrot and Apple Slices**:
   - Ingredients: Carrots, apples (cored and sliced).
   - Method: Slice carrots and apples into bite-sized pieces. Serve as crunchy and refreshing snacks that are rich in vitamins and fiber.

3. **Frozen Yogurt Drops**:
   - Ingredients: Plain yogurt, banana, blueberries.
   - Method: Blend plain yogurt with ripe banana and blueberries until smooth. Drop small spoonfuls onto a baking sheet lined with parchment paper and freeze until firm. Serve as a cool and creamy treat.

4. **Sweet Potato Chews**:
   - Ingredients: Sweet potatoes.
   - Method: Slice sweet potatoes into thin strips and bake in the oven at a low temperature until they are dehydrated and chewy. Serve as a natural and nutritious chewy treat.

5. **Chicken and Cheese Biscuits**:
   - Ingredients: Cooked chicken breast, shredded cheddar cheese,

whole wheat flour, egg.

   - Method: Mix cooked chicken breast, shredded cheddar cheese, whole wheat flour, and egg until a dough forms. Roll out the dough and cut into shapes using cookie cutters. Bake until golden brown and crispy. Serve as a protein-rich and savory snack.

6. **Frozen Fruit Popsicles**:

   - Ingredients: Assorted fruits (such as strawberries, blueberries, watermelon), coconut water.

   - Method: Chop fruits into small pieces and place them in ice cube trays. Fill the trays with coconut water and freeze until solid. Serve as a refreshing and hydrating treat on hot days.

These healthy treats and snacks are sure to delight your pup while providing them with essential nutrients and vitamins. Adjust the ingredients and portion sizes based on your dog's size and dietary needs. Always supervise your dog when giving them treats and consult with your veterinarian before introducing new foods into their diet.

Peanut Butter and Banana Biscuits Recipe:

Ingredients:
- 1 ripe banana, mashed
- 1/2 cup natural peanut butter (make sure it doesn't contain xylitol)
- 1 1/2 cups whole wheat flour
- 1 teaspoon baking powder
- 1/4 cup water (as needed)

Instructions:
1. Preheat your oven to 350°F (175°C). Line a baking sheet with parchment paper.
2. In a mixing bowl, combine the mashed banana and natural peanut butter until smooth.
3. In a separate bowl, whisk together the whole wheat flour and baking powder.
4. Gradually add the dry ingredients to the banana and peanut

butter mixture, stirring until a dough forms. If the dough is too dry, add water, a tablespoon at a time, until the dough comes together.

5. Roll out the dough on a floured surface to about 1/4 inch thickness.

6. Use cookie cutters to cut out biscuits in desired shapes.

7. Place the biscuits on the prepared baking sheet.

8. Bake in the preheated oven for 15-20 minutes, or until the biscuits are golden brown and firm to the touch.

9. Remove from the oven and let the biscuits cool completely on a wire rack.

10. Once cooled, store the peanut butter and banana biscuits in an airtight container at room temperature for up to one week.

These homemade Peanut Butter and Banana Biscuits are a delicious and wholesome treat for your pup, packed with natural flavors and nutrients. Adjust the ingredients and portion sizes based on your dog's size and dietary needs. Always supervise your dog when giving them treats and consult with your veterinarian before introducing new foods into their diet.

Carrot and Apple Pupcakes Recipe:

Ingredients:
- 1 cup whole wheat flour
- 1 teaspoon baking powder
- 1/2 cup unsweetened applesauce
- 1/4 cup honey (optional)
- 1/4 cup vegetable oil
- 1 egg
- 1/2 cup grated carrots
- 1/2 cup grated apple (cored and peeled)
- Cream cheese (optional, for frosting)

Instructions:
1. Preheat your oven to 350°F (175°C). Line a muffin tin with paper liners.
2. In a large mixing bowl, whisk together the whole wheat flour

and baking powder.

3. In a separate bowl, mix together the applesauce, honey (if using), vegetable oil, and egg until well combined.

4. Gradually add the wet ingredients to the dry ingredients, stirring until just combined.

5. Fold in the grated carrots and grated apple until evenly distributed throughout the batter.

6. Spoon the batter into the prepared muffin tin, filling each cup about 2/3 full.

7. Bake in the preheated oven for 18-20 minutes, or until the pupcakes are golden brown and a toothpick inserted into the center comes out clean.

8. Remove from the oven and let the cakes cool in the muffin tin for 5 minutes before transferring them to a wire rack to cool completely.

9. Once cooled, optionally frost the cakes with a thin layer of cream cheese.

10. Serve the carrot and apple cakes as a special treat for your pup.

These Carrot and Apple cakes are a delightful and nutritious treat for your furry friend, packed with natural sweetness and wholesome ingredients. Adjust the ingredients and portion sizes based on your dog's size and dietary needs. Always supervise your dog when giving them treats and consult with your veterinarian before introducing new foods into their diet.

Frozen Yogurt Drops Recipe:

Ingredients:
- 1 cup plain yogurt (avoid yogurt with added sugars or artificial sweeteners)
- 1 ripe banana, mashed
- 1/2 cup blueberries (fresh or frozen)

Instructions:
1. In a mixing bowl, combine the plain yogurt and mashed banana until smooth.
2. Gently fold in the blueberries until evenly distributed

throughout the mixture.

3. Line a baking sheet with parchment paper.

4. Using a spoon or a small cookie scoop, drop small dollops of the yogurt mixture onto the prepared baking sheet, spacing them apart.

5. Place the baking sheet in the freezer and freeze the yogurt drops for 1-2 hours, or until they are firm.

6. Once frozen, transfer the yogurt drops to an airtight container or freezer bag for storage.

7. Serve the frozen yogurt drops as a cool and refreshing treat for your pup.

These Frozen Yogurt Drops are a tasty and nutritious treat for your furry friend, perfect for cooling down on hot days. The combination of yogurt, banana, and blueberries provides a good source of probiotics, vitamins, and antioxidants. Adjust the ingredients and portion sizes based on your dog's size and dietary needs. Always supervise your dog when giving them treats and consult with your veterinarian before introducing new foods into their diet.

Chapter 8: Special Diets And Considerations

In this chapter, we'll explore special diets and considerations for dogs with unique dietary needs or health conditions. Whether your dog requires a specific diet due to allergies, sensitivities, or medical conditions, it's essential to tailor their meals to support their overall health and well-being.

1. **Grain-Free Diets**:
   - Some dogs may benefit from grain-free diets, especially those with grain allergies or sensitivities. Grain-free options include recipes that substitute grains with alternative sources of carbohydrates such as sweet potatoes, lentils, or peas.

2. **Limited Ingredient Diets**:
   - Dogs with food allergies or sensitivities may benefit from limited ingredient diets that contain a minimal number of ingredients. These diets typically feature a single protein source and a single carbohydrate source to reduce the risk of triggering allergic reactions.

3. **Raw Diets**:
   - Raw diets consist of uncooked meat, bones, fruits, and vegetables, mimicking the natural diet of wild canines. While some proponents believe raw diets offer health benefits such as improved coat condition and dental health, it's essential to consult with a veterinarian to ensure a balanced and safe diet.

4. **Homemade Diets for Medical Conditions**:
   - Dogs with certain medical conditions such as kidney disease, diabetes, or obesity may benefit from homemade diets tailored to their specific needs. These diets often require careful monitoring of nutrient levels and portion sizes to manage the condition effectively.

5. **Weight Management Diets**:

- Overweight or obese dogs may require weight management diets that are low in calories and fat but high in fiber and protein to promote satiety and support weight loss. These diets often involve portion control and regular exercise to achieve and maintain a healthy weight.

6. **Senior Dog Diets**:
   - Senior dogs have unique nutritional needs that may require adjustments to their diet as they age. Senior dog diets typically include lower calories, reduced fat, and increased fiber to support aging metabolism, joint health, and cognitive function.

7. **Consultation with Veterinarian or Veterinary Nutritionist**:
   - Before making significant changes to your dog's diet or implementing a special diet, it's crucial to consult with a veterinarian or veterinary nutritionist. They can provide personalized recommendations based on your dog's individual needs, health status, and dietary requirements.

By understanding special diets and considerations for dogs, you can ensure that your furry friend receives the proper nutrition and support they need to thrive. Tailoring their diet to meet their unique needs can contribute to their overall health, vitality, and longevity. Always prioritize your dog's well-being and consult with a professional for guidance on dietary decisions.

Here are two recipes suitable for dogs with allergies or sensitivities:

1. **Salmon and Sweet Potato Recipe**:

Ingredients:
- 1 lb boneless, skinless salmon fillets
- 2 sweet potatoes, peeled and diced
- 1 cup green beans, chopped
- 1 tablespoon olive oil

Instructions:
1. Preheat your oven to 375°F (190°C).

2. Place the salmon fillets on a baking sheet lined with parchment paper.

3. Drizzle the salmon with olive oil and bake for 15-20 minutes, or until cooked through.

4. While the salmon is baking, steam or boil the diced sweet potatoes and chopped green beans until tender.

5. Once the salmon is cooked, flake it into bite-sized pieces.

6. In a large mixing bowl, combine the flaked salmon, cooked sweet potatoes, and cooked green beans.

7. Mix well to combine all ingredients.

8. Allow the mixture to cool before serving to your dog.

9. Store any leftovers in an airtight container in the refrigerator for up to 3 days.

2. **Turkey and Quinoa Recipe**:

Ingredients:
- 1 lb ground turkey
- 1 cup cooked quinoa
- 1 cup carrots, shredded
- 1 cup peas (fresh or frozen)
- 1 tablespoon coconut oil (optional)

Instructions:
1. In a large skillet, cook the ground turkey over medium heat until browned and cooked through.

2. Drain any excess fat from the skillet.

3. Add cooked quinoa, shredded carrots, and peas to the skillet with the cooked turkey.

4. If using coconut oil, add it to the skillet and stir until melted and well combined.

5. Cook the mixture for an additional 5-7 minutes, or until the vegetables are tender.

6. Remove from heat and let the mixture cool before serving to your dog.

7. Store any leftovers in an airtight container in the refrigerator for up to 3 days.

These recipes are free from common allergens such as grains, dairy, and certain proteins like beef and chicken. However, it's essential to consult with your veterinarian to determine your dog's specific allergies or sensitivities and adjust the recipes accordingly.

Homemade diets for senior dogs should focus on providing balanced nutrition while considering their changing dietary needs as they age. Here's a recipe suitable for senior dogs:

Chicken and Brown Rice Stew for Senior Dogs:

Ingredients:
- 1 lb boneless, skinless chicken thighs, diced
- 1 cup brown rice
- 2 cups low-sodium chicken broth
- 1 cup carrots, diced
- 1 cup green beans, chopped
- 1/2 cup peas (fresh or frozen)
- 1 tablespoon olive oil
- 1 teaspoon dried parsley (optional, for garnish)

Instructions:
1. In a large pot, heat olive oil over medium heat. Add diced chicken thighs and cook until browned.
2. Add brown rice and chicken broth to the pot. Bring to a boil, then reduce heat to low and simmer for 15-20 minutes, or until the rice is cooked and the liquid is absorbed.
3. Add diced carrots, chopped green beans, and peas to the pot. Cook for an additional 5-7 minutes, or until the vegetables are tender.
4. Remove from heat and let the stew cool before serving to your senior dog.
5. Optionally, sprinkle dried parsley on top for garnish before serving.
6. Store any leftovers in an airtight container in the refrigerator for up to 3 days.

This homemade chicken and brown rice stew provides senior dogs with a balanced combination of lean protein, healthy carbohydrates, and essential vitamins and minerals. Adjust the ingredients and portion sizes based on your dog's size, activity level, and specific dietary needs. Additionally, consult with your veterinarian to ensure the recipe meets your senior dog's nutritional requirements and any specific health considerations they may have. Regular check-ups with the vet can help monitor your senior dog's health and adjust their diet as needed to support their overall well-being.

Tips for Overweight Dogs:

1. Controlled Portions: Measure your dog's food to ensure they are not overeating. Follow feeding guidelines provided by your veterinarian or pet food manufacturer.

2. Low-Calorie Food: Switch to a weight management or low-calorie dog food formula to help reduce calorie intake while still providing essential nutrients.

3. Increased Exercise: Incorporate regular exercise into your dog's routine. Start with short walks and gradually increase duration and intensity as your dog's fitness improves.

4. Interactive Toys: Use interactive toys or engage in active play sessions to encourage physical activity and mental stimulation.

5. Monitor Treats: Limit high-calorie treats and snacks. Instead, offer low-calorie treats such as baby carrots or green beans.

6. Regular Weigh-Ins: Monitor your dog's weight regularly and adjust their diet and exercise plan accordingly.

7. Veterinary Consultation: Consult with your veterinarian to develop a tailored weight loss plan and address any underlying health issues contributing to weight gain.

Tips for Underweight Dogs:

1. High-Calorie Diet: Choose a dog food formula with higher calorie content to help promote weight gain. Look for formulas labeled for "weight gain" or "high energy."

2. Frequent Meals: Offer frequent small meals throughout the day

to encourage eating and prevent digestive upset from large meals.

3. Nutrient-Dense Foods: Incorporate nutrient-dense foods such as lean meats, eggs, and healthy fats (e.g., coconut oil or olive oil) into your dog's diet.

4. Appetite Stimulants: Discuss appetite stimulants or supplements with your veterinarian to encourage your dog to eat.

5. Treats Between Meals: Offer high-calorie treats between meals to provide additional calories and encourage appetite.

6. Regular Veterinary Check-Ups: Schedule regular veterinary check-ups to monitor your dog's progress and adjust their diet or treatment plan as needed.

7. Address Underlying Health Issues: Rule out any underlying medical conditions that may be causing weight loss, such as gastrointestinal issues or dental problems.

Regardless of whether your dog is overweight or underweight, it's essential to consult with your veterinarian for personalized advice and guidance. They can help identify the underlying causes of your dog's weight issue and develop a tailored plan to address their specific needs. Regular veterinary check-ups can also help monitor your dog's progress and ensure they are on the right track to achieving a healthy weight.

Chapter 9: Meal Planning And Batch Cooking

In this chapter, we'll explore meal planning and batch cooking strategies to simplify the process of preparing homemade meals for your dog. By dedicating time to plan and prepare meals in advance, you can ensure that your dog receives nutritious and balanced meals while saving time and effort in the long run.

1. **Create a Weekly Meal Plan**:
   - Take some time each week to plan your dog's meals. Consider their nutritional needs, preferences, and any dietary restrictions or health considerations. Planning ahead helps ensure variety and balance in your dog's diet.

2. **Batch Cooking Sessions**:
   - Dedicate a day or two each month to batch cooking dog-friendly recipes. Prepare large quantities of meals and divide them into individual portions for easy storage and serving throughout the month.

3. **Choose Freezer-Friendly Recipes**:
   - Select recipes that freeze well and maintain their quality over time. Soups, stews, and casseroles are great options for batch cooking and freezing.

4. **Invest in Storage Containers**:
   - Invest in airtight storage containers or freezer-safe bags to store batch-cooked meals. Label containers with the date and contents for easy identification.

5. **Portion Control**:
   - Divide batch-cooked meals into individual portions suitable for your dog's size and dietary needs. This helps prevent overfeeding and ensures consistent portion sizes.

6. **Thawing and Reheating**:
   - When ready to serve, thaw frozen meals overnight in the

refrigerator or using the defrost setting on your microwave. Reheat meals as needed, ensuring they are warmed to a safe temperature before serving.

7. **Monitor Fresh Ingredients**:
   - Incorporate fresh ingredients into your dog's meals whenever possible. Consider adding fresh fruits and vegetables, lean meats, and healthy grains to provide variety and essential nutrients.

8. **Rotate Recipes**:
   - Rotate recipes regularly to prevent mealtime boredom and ensure your dog receives a diverse range of nutrients. Experiment with different ingredients and flavors to keep mealtime exciting.

By implementing meal planning and batch cooking strategies, you can streamline the process of preparing homemade meals for your dog while ensuring they receive nutritious and balanced meals tailored to their needs. With careful planning and organization, you can save time and effort while providing your dog with delicious and wholesome meals they'll love.

Creating a weekly meal plan for your dog involves careful consideration of their nutritional needs, preferences, and any dietary restrictions or health considerations they may have. Here's a sample weekly meal plan to get you started:

Day 1: Chicken And Brown Rice Stew

- Breakfast: Chicken and brown rice stew
- Dinner: Chicken and brown rice stew

Day 2: Salmon And Sweet Potato Patties

- Breakfast: Salmon and sweet potato patties
- Dinner: Salmon and sweet potato patties

Day 3: Turkey And Quinoa Casserole

- Breakfast: Turkey and quinoa casserole
- Dinner: Turkey and quinoa casserole

Day 4: Beef And Barley Stew

- Breakfast: Beef and barley stew
- Dinner: Beef and barley stew

Day 5: Chicken And Vegetable Stir-Fry

- Breakfast: Chicken and vegetable stir-fry
- Dinner: Chicken and vegetable stir-fry

Day 6: Pumpkin And Oatmeal Bake

- Breakfast: Pumpkin and oatmeal bake
- Dinner: Pumpkin and oatmeal bake

Day 7: Homemade Dog Treats

- Breakfast: Homemade dog treats
- Dinner: Homemade dog treats

This sample meal plan provides a variety of homemade recipes throughout the week, ensuring your dog receives a balanced diet with different sources of protein, carbohydrates, and vegetables. Adjust portion sizes based on your dog's size, activity level, and specific dietary needs. Additionally, consult with your veterinarian to ensure the meal plan meets your dog's nutritional requirements and any specific health considerations they may have.

Batch cooking and freezing homemade dog food is a convenient way to ensure your furry friend always has nutritious meals on hand. Here's how to do it:

1. **Choose Recipes**: Select homemade dog food recipes that freeze well and provide balanced nutrition. Recipes like stews, casseroles, and meatballs are excellent options for batch cooking.

2. **Plan Your Batch Cooking Session**: Set aside a day or weekend for batch cooking. Choose a time when you have a few hours to dedicate to preparing and cooking meals.

3. **Gather Ingredients**: Purchase all the ingredients you'll need for your chosen recipes. Make sure you have enough storage containers or freezer bags for storing the batch-cooked meals.

4. **Cook Meals in Batches**: Prepare large quantities of the recipes you've chosen. Use large pots, pans, or slow cookers to cook multiple servings at once.

5. **Cool Meals Completely**: Allow the cooked meals to cool completely before transferring them to storage containers or freezer bags. This helps prevent condensation and freezer burn.

6. **Portion Meals**: Divide the batch-cooked meals into individual

portions suitable for your dog's size and dietary needs. Label each container with the date and contents for easy identification.

7. **Freeze Meals**: Place the portioned meals in the freezer. Arrange them in a single layer if possible to allow for faster freezing. Leave some space between containers to allow for expansion.

8. **Thawing and Reheating**: When ready to serve, thaw frozen meals overnight in the refrigerator or using the defrost setting on your microwave. Reheat meals as needed, ensuring they are warmed to a safe temperature before serving.

9. **Monitor Freshness**: Keep track of the expiration dates on your frozen meals and use them within a reasonable timeframe to maintain freshness and quality.

By batch cooking and freezing homemade dog food, you can save time and ensure your dog always has access to healthy and nutritious meals. Experiment with different recipes and ingredients to keep mealtime interesting and varied for your furry friend.
Time-saving tips for busy pet parents:

1. **Meal Prep in Advance**: Spend some time on the weekend preparing meals for your pet for the upcoming week. Batch cooking and freezing meals can save time during busy weekdays.

2. **Use Automatic Feeders**: Invest in automatic pet feeders that dispense food at scheduled times. This can help ensure your pet gets their meals on time, even when you're not home.

3. **Set Up a Pet Station**: Designate an area in your home for your pet's essentials, such as food, water, toys, and grooming supplies. This makes it easy to find everything you need and saves time searching for items.

4. **Utilize Online Shopping**: Order pet supplies, food, and medications online to save time on trips to the store. Many

retailers offer auto-delivery options for recurring purchases.

5. **Create a Routine**: Establishing a consistent daily routine for feeding, exercise, and playtime can help streamline your day and make it easier to manage your pet's needs.

6. **Enlist Help**: If possible, enlist the help of family members, friends, or pet sitters to assist with pet care tasks when you're busy or away from home.

7. **Invest in Time-Saving Gadgets**: Consider investing in time-saving gadgets such as automatic litter boxes, self-cleaning pet water fountains, or interactive toys that keep pets entertained.

8. **Multitask During Walks**: Use your pet's daily walks as an opportunity to multitask. Listen to podcasts, make phone calls, or catch up on emails while you walk your pet.

9. **Simplify Grooming Routine**: Opt for low-maintenance grooming routines that require minimal time and effort. Regular brushing and nail trimming can help keep your pet's coat and nails in good condition with minimal fuss.

10. **Prioritize Quality Time**: While it's important to streamline pet care tasks, don't forget to prioritize quality time with your pet. Set aside dedicated time each day for bonding, cuddling, and playtime to strengthen your relationship.

By implementing these time-saving tips, you can streamline your pet care routine and ensure your furry friend receives the love, attention, and care they deserve, even during busy times.

Chapter 10: Beyond The Bowl: Supplementing Your Dog's Diet

In this chapter, we'll explore how to supplement your dog's diet to provide additional nutrients and support their overall health and well-being. While a balanced diet is essential, supplements can help fill nutritional gaps and address specific health concerns. Here are some key supplements to consider for your dog:

1. **Omega-3 Fatty Acids**:
   - Omega-3 fatty acids, such as those found in fish oil, are beneficial for your dog's skin, coat, joint health, and immune system. Consider adding a fish oil supplement to your dog's diet to promote healthy skin and a shiny coat, as well as to support joint health, especially in senior dogs or those with arthritis.

2. **Probiotics**:
   - Probiotics are beneficial bacteria that support digestive health and immune function. They can help maintain a healthy balance of gut flora and improve digestion, especially in dogs with sensitive stomachs or prone to digestive issues. Look for probiotic supplements specifically formulated for dogs.

3. **Joint Supplements**:
   - Joint supplements containing glucosamine, chondroitin, and MSM can help support joint health and mobility, particularly in senior dogs or breeds prone to joint problems. These supplements can help alleviate symptoms of arthritis and promote overall joint comfort and flexibility.

4. **Multivitamins**:
   - Multivitamin supplements can provide additional vitamins and minerals to fill nutritional gaps in your dog's diet. Look for supplements formulated specifically for dogs, as they contain the appropriate balance of vitamins and minerals for canine health.

5. **Antioxidants**:
   - Antioxidants, such as vitamin E, vitamin C, and selenium, help neutralize free radicals and support overall health and immune function. Consider adding antioxidant supplements to your dog's diet to promote cellular health and reduce oxidative stress.

6. **Digestive Enzymes**:
   - Digestive enzyme supplements can aid in the breakdown and absorption of nutrients, especially in dogs with digestive disorders or difficulty digesting certain foods. They can help improve nutrient absorption and alleviate symptoms of digestive upset.

7. **Herbal Supplements**:
   - Certain herbal supplements, such as chamomile, ginger, or turmeric, may have anti-inflammatory or calming properties that can benefit your dog's health. Consult with a veterinarian or holistic practitioner before introducing herbal supplements to your dog's diet.

When considering supplements for your dog, it's essential to consult with your veterinarian to determine which supplements are appropriate for your dog's individual needs and to ensure they are safe and effective. Always follow recommended dosages and guidelines provided by the manufacturer, and monitor your dog for any adverse reactions. Supplementing your dog's diet can be a valuable addition to their overall health and well-being when done thoughtfully and under the guidance of a veterinary professional.

Adding fresh fruits and vegetables to your dog's diet can provide a variety of health benefits, including essential nutrients, fiber, and antioxidants. Here are some tips for incorporating fresh fruits and vegetables into your dog's meals:

1. **Choose Dog-Safe Options**: Opt for dog-safe fruits and vegetables that are safe for your furry friend to eat. Some safe options include carrots, green beans, peas, apples (without seeds),

blueberries, bananas, and pumpkin.

2. **Introduce Gradually**: When introducing new fruits and vegetables to your dog's diet, start with small amounts and gradually increase over time. This helps prevent digestive upset and allows your dog to adjust to the new foods.

3. **Prepare Properly**: Wash and peel fruits and vegetables as needed to remove any dirt, pesticides, or bacteria. Remove seeds, pits, and cores from fruits, as these can be choking hazards or toxic to dogs.

4. **Cooked vs. Raw**: Some fruits and vegetables are best served cooked, while others can be offered raw. Cooking certain vegetables can make them easier to digest and may enhance nutrient absorption. However, some dogs enjoy crunchy raw vegetables as snacks.

5. **Serve as Treats or Meal Toppers**: Incorporate fresh fruits and vegetables into your dog's meals as healthy snacks or meal toppers. You can mix them into your dog's regular food or serve them as standalone treats.

6. **Monitor Portion Sizes**: Be mindful of portion sizes when feeding fruits and vegetables to your dog. While they offer health benefits, they should be given in moderation to prevent overfeeding and maintain a balanced diet.

7. **Avoid Toxic Foods**: Avoid feeding your dog toxic fruits and vegetables, such as grapes, raisins, onions, garlic, and avocados. These foods can be harmful or even deadly to dogs and should be avoided entirely.

8. **Consult with Your Veterinarian**: Before introducing new fruits and vegetables to your dog's diet, consult with your veterinarian, especially if your dog has any underlying health conditions or dietary restrictions.

Incorporating fresh fruits and vegetables into your dog's diet can add variety and nutrition to their meals while promoting overall health and well-being. With proper preparation and moderation, fruits and vegetables can be a delicious and nutritious addition to your furry friend's diet.

Incorporating supplements for joint health and shiny coats into your dog's diet can provide additional support for their overall well-being. Here are some tips for incorporating these supplements:

1. **Joint Health Supplements**:
   - Choose supplements containing ingredients such as glucosamine, chondroitin, MSM (methylsulfonylmethane), and omega-3 fatty acids.
   - Look for joint health supplements specifically formulated for dogs, available in various forms such as chewable tablets, soft chews, or liquid formulations.
   - Administer the recommended dosage based on your dog's size, age, and specific joint health needs.
   - Introduce joint health supplements gradually into your dog's diet and monitor for any adverse reactions.
   - Consider consulting with your veterinarian before starting any new joint health supplement regimen, especially if your dog has existing joint issues or is taking other medications.

2. **Omega-3 Fatty Acid Supplements**:
   - Choose supplements containing high-quality fish oil, which is rich in omega-3 fatty acids such as EPA (eicosapentaenoic acid) and DHA (docosahexaenoic acid).
   - Omega-3 fatty acids support joint health, reduce inflammation, and promote healthy skin and coat.
   - Look for fish oil supplements specifically formulated for dogs, available in liquid or capsule form.
   - Administer the recommended dosage based on your dog's size and weight.
   - Incorporate omega-3 fatty acid supplements into your dog's daily diet by mixing them with their food or administering them

directly.

3. **Incorporating Supplements into Meals**:
   - Mix joint health supplements or omega-3 fatty acid supplements with your dog's regular meals to ensure they consume them consistently.
   - If your dog is reluctant to eat supplements mixed with their food, consider using pill pockets, treat balls, or other methods to disguise the supplements and make them more palatable.

4. **Monitor Progress**:
   - Regularly monitor your dog's joint health and coat condition after incorporating supplements into their diet.
   - Look for improvements in mobility, joint stiffness, coat shine, and skin health.
   - Adjust the dosage or type of supplement as needed based on your dog's response and any recommendations from your veterinarian.

Incorporating supplements for joint health and shiny coats into your dog's diet can help support their overall health and vitality. With proper administration and monitoring, these supplements can contribute to your dog's well-being and quality of life.
Homemade remedies can provide natural relief for common health issues in dogs. Here are some homemade remedies for a few common health concerns:

1. **Skin Irritations and Hot Spots**:
   - Apple Cider Vinegar Solution: Mix equal parts of apple cider vinegar and water in a spray bottle. Apply the solution to affected areas of the skin to soothe irritation and reduce inflammation.
   - Oatmeal Bath: Prepare a warm bath with colloidal oatmeal (finely ground oatmeal) mixed into the water. Soak your dog in the oatmeal bath for 10-15 minutes to relieve itching and irritation.

2. **Upset Stomach**:
   - Plain Yogurt: Plain yogurt with live active cultures can help soothe an upset stomach and restore balance to the digestive

system. Offer a small amount of plain yogurt as a treat or mix it with your dog's food.

- Plain Boiled Chicken and Rice: Boil plain chicken breast and plain white rice without seasoning. Feed small portions of this bland diet to your dog to settle their stomach and provide easy-to-digest nutrition.

3. **Bad Breath**:

- Parsley Sprinkle: Fresh parsley contains chlorophyll, which can help freshen your dog's breath. Chop fresh parsley and sprinkle a small amount over your dog's food as a natural breath freshener.

- Coconut Oil: Add a small amount of coconut oil to your dog's food or rub it on their teeth and gums to help reduce bacteria and improve oral health.

4. **Fleas and Ticks**:

- Apple Cider Vinegar Flea Spray: Mix equal parts of apple cider vinegar and water in a spray bottle. Spritz your dog's coat with the solution, avoiding the eyes and nose, to repel fleas and ticks.

- Homemade Flea Collar: Add a few drops of essential oils such as lavender, cedarwood, or lemongrass to your dog's collar to repel fleas and ticks naturally. Make sure to dilute essential oils properly and avoid using them on sensitive dogs or puppies.

5. **Anxiety and Stress**:

- Lavender Aromatherapy: Diffuse lavender essential oil in your home or apply a few drops to your dog's bedding to promote relaxation and reduce anxiety.

- Thundershirt: Wrap your dog in a snug-fitting Thundershirt or similar anxiety-reducing garment to provide comfort and security during stressful situations.

Remember to consult with your veterinarian before trying any homemade remedies, especially if your dog has underlying health conditions or if symptoms persist. While these remedies can provide temporary relief for mild issues, professional veterinary care may be necessary for more serious or chronic conditions.

Epilogue:

As we come to the end of this journey through the world of homemade dog food, I am filled with gratitude for the opportunity to share this information with you. Throughout these pages, we have explored the importance of nutrition in supporting the health and well-being of our canine companions, and we have delved into the benefits of preparing homemade meals tailored to your dog's specific needs.

I hope this book has empowered you to take control of your dog's diet and provide them with the nourishment they deserve. Whether you choose to follow the recipes provided here or use them as inspiration to create your own culinary masterpieces, the most important thing is that you are making informed choices that prioritize your dog's health and happiness.

As we move forward, let us continue to advocate for the well-being of our furry friends and strive to provide them with the love, care, and nutrition they need to thrive. Together, we can create a world where every dog receives the best possible care and lives a long, healthy, and fulfilling life.

Thank you for joining me on this journey, and may your bond with your canine companion grow stronger with each homemade meal shared.

With warmest wishes,

[Kenneth Christopher]

Summary:

In this book, we embarked on a journey to explore the world of homemade dog food and holistic pet care. We began by understanding the nutritional needs of dogs and the importance of balanced meals for optimal health. Along the way, we debunked common misconceptions about dog food ingredients and compared homemade versus commercial options.

We delved into the kitchen essentials and safe food handling practices necessary for preparing homemade dog food, as well as tips for storing meals to maintain freshness and quality. Building upon this foundation, we discussed the role of protein, carbohydrates, fats, vitamins, and minerals in canine nutrition, along with recommended ratios for different life stages and breeds.

Next, we explored a variety of meaty marvels, carb creations, and healthy treats and snacks to add variety and nutrition to your dog's diet. From chicken stews to quinoa bakes and peanut butter biscuits, there's something for every furry friend's palate.

We also discussed special diets and considerations, including recipes for dogs with allergies or sensitivities, as well as homemade remedies for common health issues such as skin irritations, upset stomachs, and bad breath.

Throughout this journey, we emphasized the importance of dedication and acknowledgement in providing the best possible care for our canine companions. By incorporating supplements for joint health and shiny coats, as well as dedicating ourselves to their well-being, we can ensure our dogs lead happy, healthy lives filled with love and nourishment.

As we conclude our exploration, let us continue to prioritize the health and happiness of our furry friends, sharing in the joy and companionship they bring to our lives each and every day.

With warm regards,

[Kenneth Christopher]